Breaking Through the Clouds:

A Guide to Overcoming Postpartum Depression

Kathleen Bray

TABLE OF CONTENT

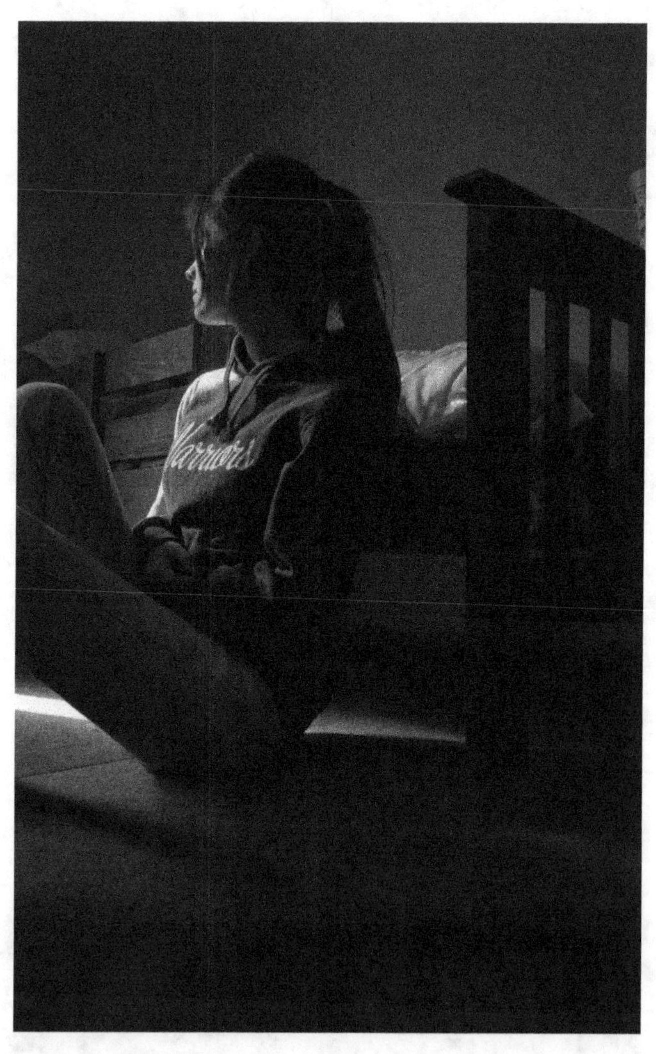

Warriors

Introduction

In the symphony of motherhood, where the world expects joyous crescendos and harmonious melodies, there exists a haunting note that often goes unheard—the disquieting tune of postpartum depression. While the arrival of a new life is meant to be a euphoric crescendo, for many mothers, it unfolds against a backdrop of silent struggles and unspoken battles.

Postpartum depression, an elusive spectre that weaves its way into the fabric of maternal joy, is a force that demands acknowledgement, understanding, and compassion. It's not a fleeting moment of melancholy but a profound and persistent storm that can cloud the brightest days with shadows of despair.

This guide delves into the complexities of postpartum depression, unravelling its nuances and shedding light on the myriad ways it can impact the lives of new mothers. We embark on a journey through the highs and lows of this emotional landscape, recognizing the importance of compassion, support, and a collective effort to bring this silent struggle into the open.

In the following pages, we explore the depths of postpartum depression, but more importantly, we navigate the pathways to resilience, recovery, and rediscovery of joy. Let this guide be a beacon for those navigating the storm, a testament to the strength within, and a reminder that, even in the darkest moments, there is a way to find the light.

Chapter One

Overview of Postpartum Depression

Postpartum depression is an intricate tapestry of emotional challenges that can shroud the initial days, weeks, or even months following childbirth. Postpartum depression is a psychiatric disorder marked by persistent feelings of melancholy, anxiety, and overwhelming weariness, much beyond the fleeting emotional changes commonly attributed to the **"baby blues."** It can manifest in various forms, affecting not only the emotional well-being of the new mother but also her physical health and ability to engage in daily activities.

An overwhelming sense of grief, altered sleep patterns, a loss of interest in activities, feelings of guilt or worthlessness, and, in extreme situations, thoughts of harming oneself or the unborn child are some of the symptoms of postpartum depression. It is a silent struggle that, more often than not, goes unrecognized, underscoring the need for heightened awareness and understanding.

Importance of Addressing Postpartum Depression

Addressing postpartum depression is not just a matter of emotional well-being; it is a critical component of maternal and family health. The impacts of untreated postpartum depression extend beyond the individual, influencing the dynamics of relationships and the overall family environment. For the mother, it can impede the bonding process with the newborn, disrupt daily functioning, and cast a long shadow over what should be a time of joy and connection.

Moreover, untreated postpartum depression can have lasting effects on the developmental trajectory of the child. Research suggests that the emotional well-being of the mother is intricately linked to the child's cognitive and emotional development. In addition to assisting the mother on her road to recovery, diagnosing and treating postpartum depression also helps to create a stable and caring environment for the entire family.

In the subsequent sections, we delve deeper into the nuances of postpartum depression, exploring its various facets and offering insights into effective strategies for identification, management, and recovery It is a call to action, requiring everyone to

collaborate to eradicate the stigma attached to
postpartum depression and establish a helpful,
comprehending, and compassionate environment
for the mothers navigating this complex terrain.

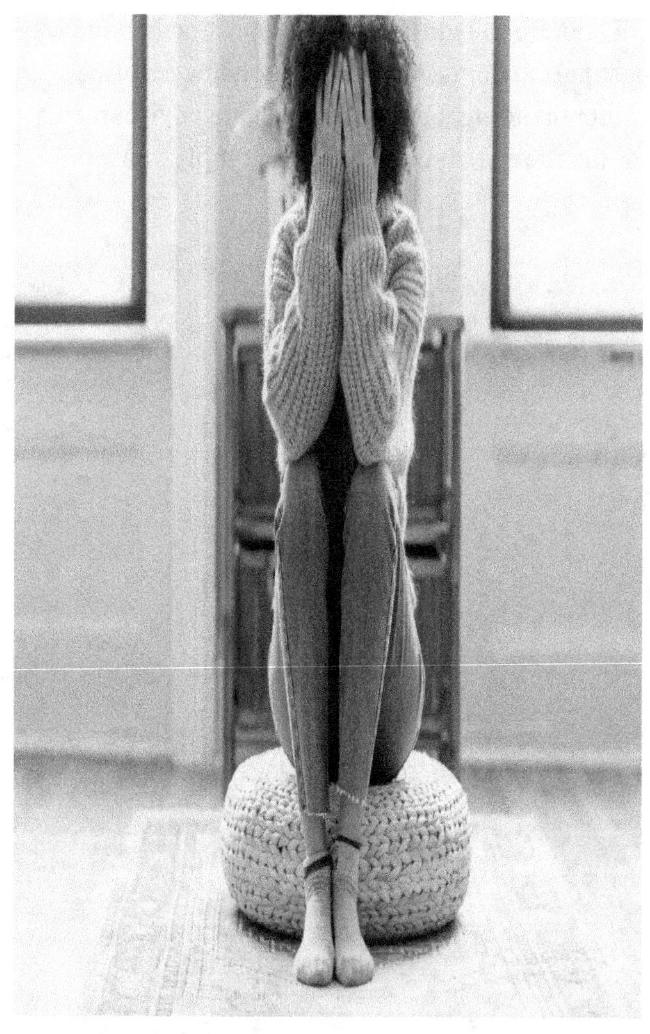

Chapter Two

Understanding Postpartum Depression

Definition and Symptoms

Postpartum depression is a multifaceted mental health condition that affects individuals after childbirth. It transcends the transient emotional fluctuations commonly known as the "baby blues" and manifests as a more persistent and intense form of depression. The symptoms of postpartum depression encompass a broad spectrum of emotional and physical challenges. These may include:

- **Persistent Sadness:** A deep and enduring feeling of sadness that persists over an extended period.
- **Fatigue:** Overwhelming fatigue and a sense of profound exhaustion, often unrelated to the physical demands of caring for a newborn.
- **Changes in Sleep Patterns:** Disruptions in sleep, either through insomnia or excessive sleeping.

- **Diminished Interest:** A decrease in the enjoyment or interest in once-pleasurable activities.
- **Feelings of Guilt or Worthlessness:** Experiencing unwarranted guilt, feelings of worthlessness, or a heightened sense of inadequacy.
- **Difficulty bonding with the Baby:** Challenges forming a strong emotional connection with the newborn.

Causes and Risk Factors

The origins of postpartum depression are complex and multifactorial, involving a combination of biological, psychological, and social factors. Some of the contributing causes and risk factors include:

- **Hormonal Change:** Hormonal variations may play a role in postpartum depression. One such fluctuation is an abrupt fall in progesterone and estrogen after childbirth.
- **History of Mental Health Issues:** A personal or family history of mental health disorders, especially depression or anxiety, can increase the likelihood of experiencing postpartum depression.
- **Stressful Life Events:** Major life stressors, such as relationship problems, financial

difficulties, or major life transformations, can cause postpartum depression.
- **Lack of Social Support:** Insufficient support from partners, family, or friends can amplify the challenges faced by new mothers.
- **Unplanned Pregnancy:** Unplanned or unwanted pregnancies may increase the risk of postpartum depression.

Prevalence and Statistics

Postpartum depression is a prevalent and global concern, affecting women across cultural, socioeconomic, and geographic boundaries. While estimates vary, it is generally reported that around 10-15% of mothers experience postpartum depression. However, due to underreporting and the stigma associated with mental health, the actual prevalence may be higher.

It's essential to recognise that postpartum depression can affect any woman, regardless of age, race, or socioeconomic status. By understanding the definition, symptoms, causes, and risk factors, we can begin to dismantle the barriers that prevent timely recognition and intervention, fostering an environment that promotes the well-being of new mothers.

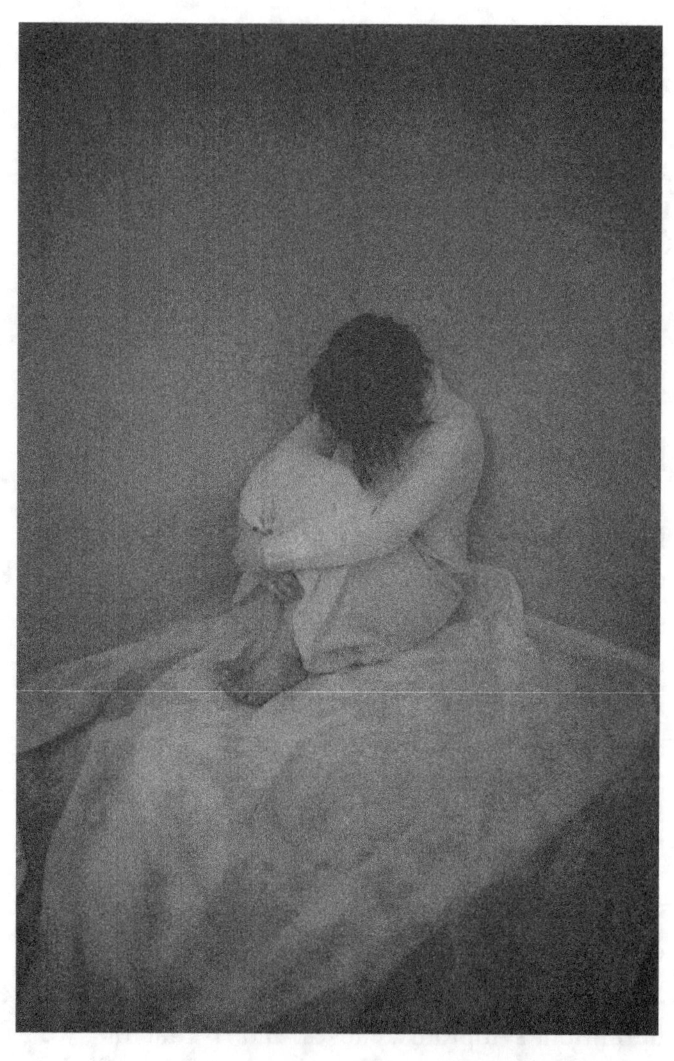

Chapter Three

Identifying Postpartum Depression

Signs and Symptoms

As mentioned in the last chapter, several behavioural, physical, and emotional indicators can indicate postpartum depression. Though every person's experience is unique, typical indications and symptoms consist of:

1. **Persistent Sadness:** Overwhelming and enduring feelings of sadness or emptiness.
2. **Extreme Fatigue:** A pervasive sense of exhaustion, even after rest or sleep.
3. **Changes in Sleep Patterns:** Disruptions in sleep, either difficulty sleeping or excessive sleeping.
4. **Appetite Changes:** Significant alterations in appetite, leading to weight loss or gain.
5. **Difficulty bonding with the Baby:** Struggles to form a strong emotional connection with the newborn.
6. **Loss of Interest or Pleasure:** Diminished interest in activities that were once enjoyable or fulfilling.

7. **Feelings of Worthlessness or Guilt:** Unwarranted feelings of inadequacy, guilt, or hopelessness.
8. **Difficulty Concentrating:** Challenges in focusing, making decisions, or completing tasks.
9. **Irritability or Anger:** Increased irritability, frustration, or even anger without apparent cause.
10. **Physical Symptoms:** Ailments like headaches or stomach aches without a clear medical explanation.

It's important to note that experiencing some of these symptoms is not uncommon in the early postpartum period. However, when these symptoms persist, intensify, or significantly impair daily functioning, it may be indicative of postpartum depression.

Differentiating Between "Baby Blues" and Postpartum Depression

Baby Blues:

- **Onset:** Typically within the first few days after childbirth.
- **Duration:** Resolves within the first two weeks.

- **Intensity:** Mild mood swings, occasional weepiness, and general feelings of being overwhelmed.

Postpartum Depression:

- **Onset:** Can occur at any time within the first year after childbirth.
- **Duration:** Symptoms persist beyond the initial two weeks, often for months.
- **Intensity:** More intense and enduring symptoms that interfere with daily functioning and well-being.

- ❖ It's crucial to recognize the duration, intensity, and impact of symptoms. If a mother experiences persistent and debilitating feelings, reaching out for professional support and guidance becomes essential. Efficient identification and effective management of postpartum depression necessitate candid communication between partners, medical experts, and support networks.

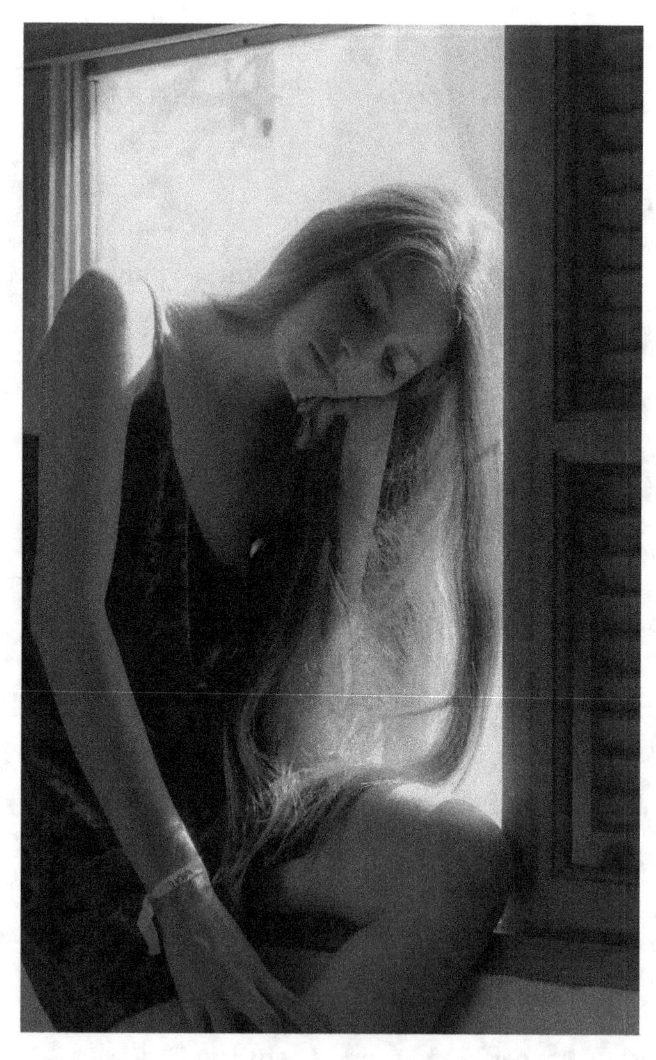

Chapter Four

Effects of Postpartum Depression

Postpartum depression (PPD) is a complex and challenging condition that affects mothers after childbirth. Its effects extend beyond the individual, influencing family dynamics and relationships, and may have long-term consequences. Understanding these impacts is crucial for providing support and intervention.

Impact on Mothers:

1. **Emotional Turmoil:** Postpartum depression can lead to intense feelings of sadness, despair, and hopelessness for mothers. The joy and excitement commonly associated with childbirth are often overshadowed by persistent negative emotions.

2. **Physical Symptoms:** PPD may manifest physically, contributing to fatigue, changes in appetite, and disturbances in sleep patterns. The physical toll can exacerbate the emotional strain, making it challenging for mothers to care for themselves and their infants.

3. **Bonding Issues:** Mothers experiencing PPD may find it difficult to bond with their newborns. This lack of connection can impact the development of a healthy parent-child relationship and may hinder the establishment of a secure attachment.
4. **Shame and guilt:** Mothers with PPD often experience feelings of shame and guilt, believing that they are failing as parents. This emotional burden can perpetuate the cycle of depression and hinder the ability to seek help.

Impact on Family and Relationships:

1. **Strained Partner Relationships:** PPD can strain relationships with partners. The emotional distance and mood changes may lead to misunderstandings, increased tension, and strained communication.
2. **Parenting Challenges:** The family dynamic can be disrupted as the affected mother may struggle with daily parenting responsibilities. This can place additional stress on the partner and impact the overall functioning of the family unit.
3. **Impact on Siblings:** If there are older siblings, they may be affected by the changes in the mother's mood and behaviour. The household atmosphere may

become tense, impacting the emotional well-being of all family members.

4. **Social Isolation:** Mothers with PPD may withdraw from social activities, leading to isolation from friends and extended family. This can further exacerbate feelings of loneliness and contribute to the overall strain on relationships.

Long-Term Consequences:

1. **Child Developmental Outcomes:** PPD has been linked to long-term effects on child development. Children born to mothers with untreated PPD may be at an increased risk of behavioural and emotional problems, as well as cognitive delays.

2. **Recurrence Risk:** Women who experience PPD are at a higher risk of recurrence with subsequent pregnancies. Recognizing and addressing PPD early is crucial to break this cycle and minimize the impact on both the mother and the family.

3. **Impact on Maternal Mental Health:** Untreated postpartum depression (PPD) can take a mother's lifetime to heal, which raises the possibility that she will have chronic depression. Seeking timely intervention is essential for preventing long-term consequences.

4. **Inter-generational Impact:** The effects of
   PPD can transcend generations. It is crucial
   to interrupt the cycle of mental health issues
   in children whose moms had PPD by
   providing early intervention and support, as
   this may raise the kids' chance of developing
   mental health issues as adults.

* The effects of postpartum depression are
  multifaceted, impacting not only the mother
  but also the entire family unit. Recognizing
  the signs, providing support, and seeking
  professional help are essential components
  of mitigating the short and long-term
  consequences associated with PPD.

Chapter Five

Seeking Professional Help

Seeking professional help is a crucial step for individuals experiencing mental health challenges, including conditions like postpartum depression (PPD). Professional support can provide valuable guidance, coping strategies, and interventions to promote recovery and well-being.

Importance of Professional Support:

1. **Expertise and Training:**
   - Mental health professionals possess the education, training, and expertise to understand and address the complexities of postpartum depression. They can diagnose the condition, assess its severity, and tailor interventions to individual needs.

2. **Objective Perspective:**
   - Professionals offer an unbiased and objective perspective, providing a safe space for individuals to express their thoughts and feelings without fear of judgment. Understanding the

fundamental causes of postpartum depression and developing successful treatment regimens require this perspective.

3. **Specialized Knowledge:**
4. Psychologists, psychiatrists, and licensed therapists are among the mental health professionals who frequently have specialized training in perinatal mental health to manage the unique challenges associated with postpartum depression.
5. **Medication Management:**
   - In cases where medication is deemed necessary, psychiatrists can prescribe and monitor medication to alleviate symptoms. They work collaboratively with individuals to find the most suitable treatment options, considering potential benefits and side effects.
6. **Therapeutic Alliance:**
   - Building a therapeutic alliance with a mental health professional fosters a supportive and trusting relationship. This connection can be a vital component of the healing process, helping individuals feel understood, validated, and empowered to make positive changes.

Types of Mental Health Professionals:

1. **Psychiatrist:**
   - Medical professionals with a focus on mental health are called psychiatrists. They can diagnose mental health conditions, prescribe medication, and provide a comprehensive approach to treatment.
2. **Psychologist:**
   - Psychologists hold advanced degrees in psychology and use therapeutic techniques to help individuals understand and manage their thoughts, emotions, and behaviours. They can offer various types of therapy.
3. **Licensed Counsellor or Therapist:**
   - Licensed counsellors or therapists have specialized training in providing talk therapy. For those suffering from postpartum depression, they can provide support, direction, and coping mechanisms.
4. **Social Worker:**
   - Clinical social workers with mental health training can provide counselling and support. They may

also assist individuals in navigating social and community resources.

5. **Perinatal Mental Health Specialist:**
   - Some mental health professionals specialize in perinatal mental health, focusing on issues related to pregnancy, childbirth, and the postpartum period. They are well-versed in addressing conditions like postpartum depression.

Therapy Options:

1. **Cognitive-Behavioural Therapy (CBT):**
   - CBT is a popular therapy strategy that assists patients in recognizing and altering unfavourable thought and behaviour patterns. It can be effective in treating postpartum depression by addressing distorted thinking and promoting healthier coping strategies.
2. **Interpersonal Therapy (IPT):**
   - IPT is centred on enhancing communication and interpersonal skills. It is particularly useful for individuals experiencing difficulties in their relationships due to postpartum depression.
3. **Supportive Psychotherapy:**

- o Supportive psychotherapy provides a safe space for individuals to express their emotions and concerns while receiving guidance and support from the therapist.

4. **Medication Management:**
   - o Psychiatrists may recommend medications, including antidepressants, to treat postpartum depression symptoms. Medication and therapy are frequently used for a holistic approach to treatment.

5. **Group Therapy:**
   - o Group therapy involves individuals with similar challenges coming together to share their experiences, provide mutual support, and learn coping strategies under the guidance of a trained therapist.

❖ Seeking professional help is a proactive and empowering step towards managing postpartum depression. The collaborative efforts of mental health professionals and individuals experiencing PPD can lead to effective treatment, symptom relief, and a pathway to improved mental health and well-being. It's important to remember that reaching out for support is a sign of strength, and there are resources available to assist in the journey towards recovery.

Chapter Six

Self-Help Strategies

The use of self-help techniques is essential for controlling and reducing postpartum depression (PPD) symptoms. These strategies empower individuals to actively participate in their well-being and complement professional interventions. Here are key self-help strategies for individuals experiencing PPD:

1. Building a Support System:
- **Connect with Loved Ones:** Share your thoughts and feelings with trusted friends, family members, or a partner. Establishing open communication can help reduce feelings of isolation.
- **Join Support Groups:** Participate in local or online support groups for mothers experiencing postpartum depression. Sharing experiences with others who can relate can provide a sense of understanding and community.
- **Delegate Responsibilities:** Don't hesitate to ask for help with daily tasks. Whether it's childcare, household chores, or errands,

delegating responsibilities can ease the burden and create space for self-care.

2. Self-Care Practices:
- **Make sleep a priority:** Try to get enough good sleep. Develop a bedtime routine, create a comfortable sleep environment, and enlist the help of others to care for the baby during the night.
- **Healthy Nutrition:** Maintain a balanced and nutritious diet to support physical and mental well-being. Ensure you're getting essential nutrients, and stay hydrated.
- **Regular Exercise:** Engage in gentle exercises, such as walking or yoga, to promote the release of endorphins and boost mood. See a medical professional before beginning a new fitness regimen.
- **Mindfulness and Relaxation Techniques:** Practice mindfulness, deep breathing, or meditation to manage stress and stay grounded. To encourage a sense of calm, these methods might be added to regular activities.

3. Managing Stress:
- **Set Realistic Expectations:** Adjust expectations and recognize that it's okay if everything doesn't go as planned Prioritize

what is most important and set attainable goals.

- **Time Management:** Break tasks into smaller, more manageable steps. Create a schedule that allows for breaks and self-care, avoiding overwhelming commitments.
- **Know When to Say No:** It's important to know your boundaries. Politely decline additional responsibilities or commitments that may contribute to stress and overwhelm.

4. Enhancing Sleep Quality:

- **Establish a Routine:** Create a bedtime routine that signals to your body that it's time to wind down. Reading a book or having a warm bath are two examples of this.
- **Create a Comfortable Sleep Environment:** Ensure your bedroom is conducive to sleep by maintaining a cool, dark, and quiet environment. Spend money on a supportive mattress and cosy bedding.
- **Limit Screen Time:** Reduce exposure to screens before bedtime, as the blue light emitted can interfere with melatonin production and disrupt sleep.

5. Journaling and Reflection:

- **Express Emotions:** Use journaling as a tool to express your thoughts and emotions. Writing down your feelings can provide clarity and serve as a means of self-reflection.
- **Celebrate Achievements:** Acknowledge and celebrate small victories, no matter how minor. Recognizing accomplishments, even daily, can boost self-esteem.

6. Mindful Parenting:

- **Focus on the Present Moment:** Practice mindful parenting by staying present with your child. Engage in activities together, paying attention to the sights, sounds, and emotions of the moment.
- **Seek Joyful Moments:** Look for and savour moments of joy and connection with your child. These positive experiences can contribute to an overall sense of well-being.

- ❖ Incorporating self-help strategies into daily life is a valuable and proactive approach to managing postpartum depression. These practices, when combined with professional support, contribute to a holistic and effective treatment plan. Remember that self-care is

not selfish but rather an essential aspect of
maintaining mental and emotional health
during the challenging postpartum period.

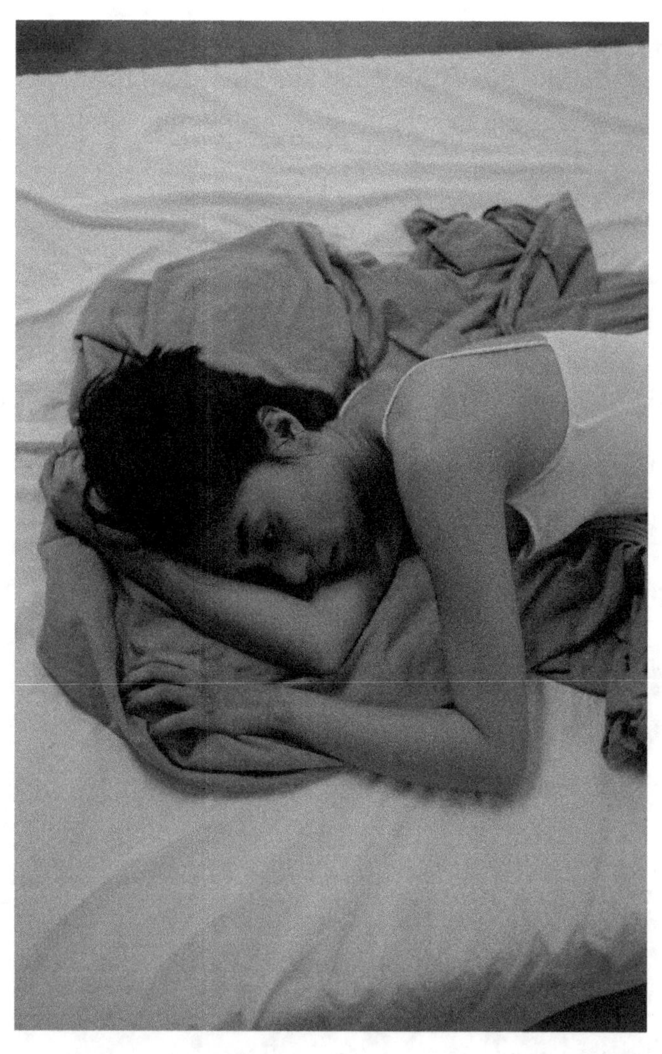

Chapter Seven

Medical Interventions

Medical interventions, particularly medications, can be a vital component of the treatment plan for postpartum depression (PPD). It's important to note that medication decisions should be made in consultation with a healthcare professional, taking into account individual circumstances, the severity of symptoms, and potential risks and benefits.

Medications for Postpartum Depression:

1. **Antidepressants:**
   - **Selective Serotonin Reuptake Inhibitors (SSRIs):** SSRIs, such as fluoxetine (Prozac) and sertraline (Zoloft), are commonly prescribed for PPD. They work by increasing the levels of serotonin in the brain, improving mood and reducing depressive symptoms.
   - **Serotonin-Norepinephrine Reuptake Inhibitors (SNRIs):** Medications like venlafaxine (Effexor) may be considered. SNRIs affect both serotonin and norepinephrine levels in the brain.

2. **Atypical Antidepressants:**
   - **Bupropion (Wellbutrin):** This medication works on norepinephrine and dopamine levels and may be considered as an alternative in some cases.
3. **Hormone Therapy:**
   - **Estrogen Replacement Therapy:** Some studies suggest that estrogen may play a role in the development of PPD, and hormone therapy may be considered in certain cases. However, this approach is not universally accepted and has its own set of considerations and risks.

Potential Side Effects and Considerations:

1. **Side Effects:**
   - **Common Side Effects:** Antidepressants may cause side effects, including nausea, insomnia, weight changes, and sexual dysfunction. It's crucial to communicate openly with the healthcare provider about any side effects experienced.

- **Activation or Agitation:** Some individuals may experience increased anxiety or agitation when starting an antidepressant. Monitoring for these symptoms is essential.

2. **Delayed Onset of Action:**
   - It frequently takes several weeks for antidepressants to fully take action. Patience is crucial during this period, and individuals should be informed that improvement may not be immediate.

3. **Adjustment of Medication:**
   - Finding the right medication and dosage may involve a trial-and-error process. It's not uncommon for healthcare providers to make adjustments based on the individual's response and side effects.

4. **Considerations for Breastfeeding:**
   - Many antidepressants pass into breast milk, so the decision to use medication while breastfeeding requires careful consideration. Healthcare providers can help assess the risks and benefits and explore options that are safer for breastfeeding.

5. **Monitoring for Suicidal Thoughts:**
   - Antidepressants are generally safe, but in some cases, they may initially increase the risk of suicidal thoughts. Close monitoring, especially during the early stages of treatment, is essential.
6. **Interaction with Other Medications:**
   - Inform the healthcare provider about any other medications, including over-the-counter drugs and herbal supplements, to avoid potential interactions.
7. **Relapse Prevention:**
   - Frequently, doctors prescribe medication for a set amount of time. It's essential to follow the prescribed treatment plan and not discontinue medication abruptly. Discontinuation should be done under the guidance of a healthcare professional to minimize the risk of relapse.
8. **Communication with Healthcare Provider:**
   - Open and honest communication with the healthcare provider is critical. If any concerns or side effects arise, it's important to discuss them promptly to make informed

decisions about the course of
treatment.

❖   Medications can be effective in treating
postpartum depression, but they are not a
one-size-fits-all solution. Each individual's
situation is unique, and the decision to use
medication should be made collaboratively
between the individual and their healthcare
provider. Regular monitoring, open
communication, and a comprehensive
treatment plan that may include therapy and
support are key elements in addressing
postpartum depression effectively.

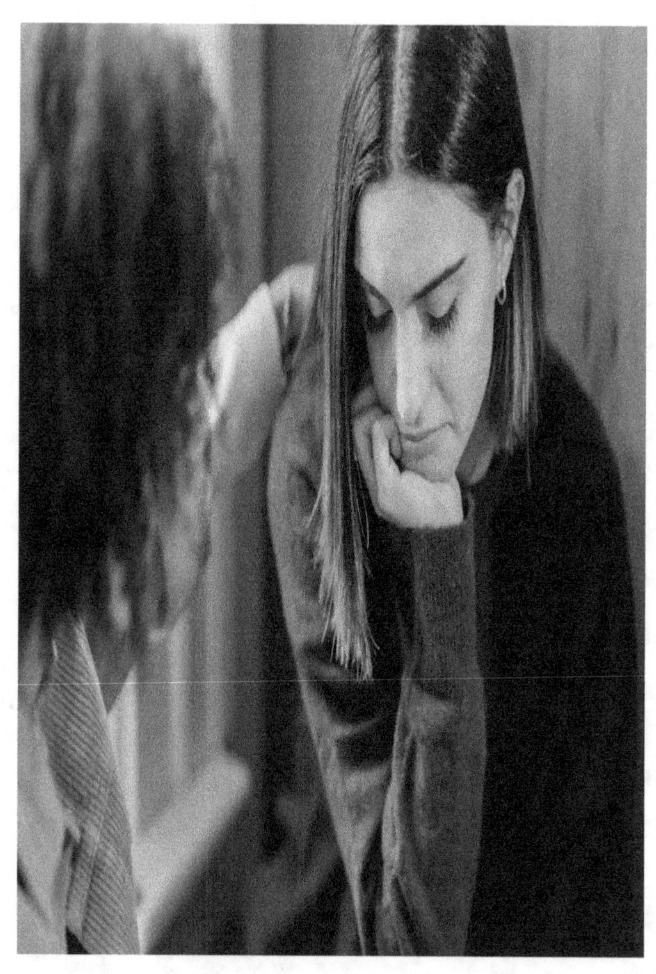

Chapter Eight

Counselling and Support Groups

Counselling and support groups are crucial places to go for therapeutic therapies and emotional support for those with postpartum depression (PPD). These avenues offer unique benefits that contribute to the overall well-being of those grappling with this challenging condition.

Benefits of Counseling for Postpartum Depression:

1. **Professional Guidance:**
   - **Expert Insight:** Counsellors, therapists, and mental health professionals have specialized training in addressing mental health issues, including postpartum depression. They offer expert guidance and insights to help individuals navigate their emotions and challenges.
2. **Individualized Support:**

3. **Tailored Interventions:** Counseling allows for personalized treatment plans based on the specific needs and circumstances of the individual. Therapists might adapt their methods to meet the unique factors that lead to postpartum depression.

4. **Safe and Confidential Space:**
   - **Non-Judgmental Environment:** Counseling sessions provide a safe and confidential space where individuals can express their thoughts, feelings, and concerns without fear of judgment. This encourages open communication and self-reflection.

5. **Coping Strategies:**
   - **Improvement of Skills:** Through counselling, people can learn useful coping mechanisms and techniques to handle their stress, feelings, and the difficulties associated with postpartum depression. These skills empower individuals to actively work towards their well-being.

6. **Relationship Enhancement:**
   - **Improving Communication:** For individuals dealing with strained relationships due to **PPD**, counselling can help improve

communication and understanding
between partners and family
members. It fosters a collaborative
approach to coping with the effects
of postpartum depression.

Participating in Support Groups for Postpartum Depression:

1. **Validation and Empathy:**
   - **Feeling Understood:** Being part of a support group provides validation and empathy. Sharing experiences with others who have gone through or are going through similar challenges helps individuals feel understood and less alone.
2. **Practical Advice:**
   - **Learning from Others:** Support groups offer a platform for sharing practical advice and tips for managing day-to-day challenges associated with PPD. Participants can learn from each other's coping strategies.
3. **Normalization of Feelings:**
   - **Identifying Common Experiences:** Learning about other people's

experiences in a support group can help postpartum depression-related feelings and experiences seem more normal. This normalization reduces the stigma often attached to mental health conditions.

4. **Peer Support:**
   - **Encouragement and Validation:** Participants in support groups provide encouragement and validation to one another. This peer support can be a powerful motivator for seeking help, adhering to treatment plans, and making positive changes.

5. **Building Social Connections:**
   - **Forming Friendships:** Support groups offer an opportunity to build social connections. Forming friendships with individuals who understand the challenges of postpartum depression can contribute to a strong support network.

❖ Counseling and support groups are valuable resources for individuals experiencing postpartum depression. Whether through individual therapy sessions or group settings, these avenues provide a combination of professional guidance, emotional support, and shared experiences that contribute to the holistic approach to recovery. Combining these supportive interventions with other treatment modalities, such as medication and self-help strategies, can lead to more comprehensive and effective management of postpartum depression.

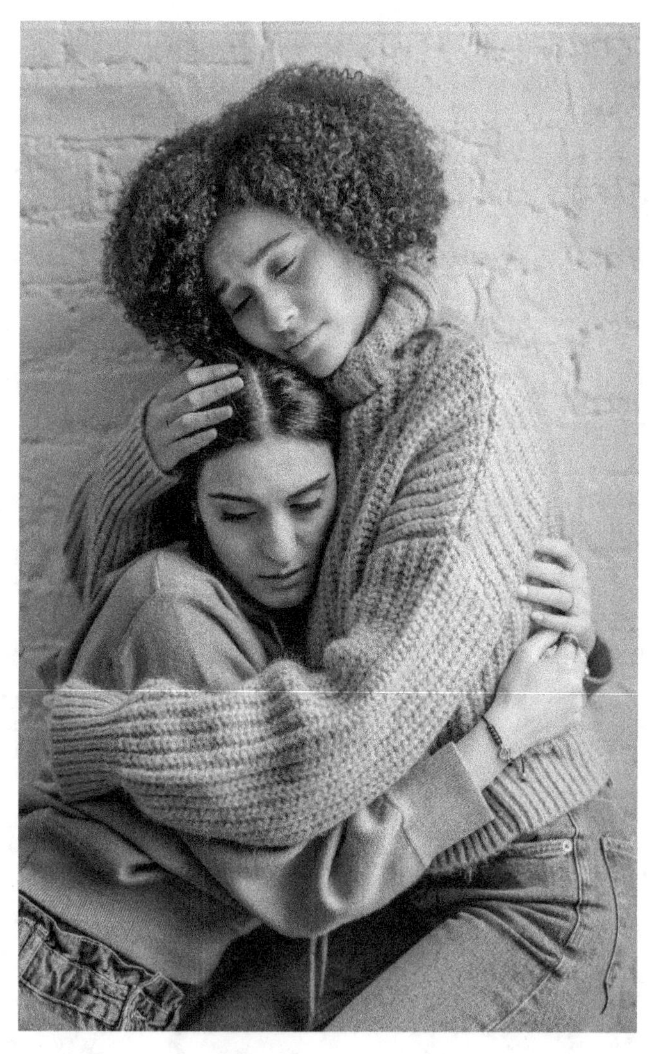

Chapter Nine

Partner and Family Support

Support from partners and family is essential during the recovery process for those with postpartum depression (PPD). Open communication, understanding, and active involvement of loved ones can significantly contribute to the overall well-being of the individual and the family unit.

Communicating with Partners and Family:

1. **Open Dialogue:**
   - **Expressing Feelings:** Individuals experiencing PPD should communicate openly with their partners and family members about their thoughts, emotions, and challenges. This open dialogue fosters understanding and establishes a foundation for support.
2. **Educating Partners and Family:**
   - **Sharing Information:** Provide partners and family members with information about postpartum depression, including its symptoms and potential impact. Education can

help loved ones better understand the condition and respond empathetically.

3. **Setting Realistic Expectations:**
    - **Managing Expectations:** Establish realistic expectations for recovery and acknowledge that healing may take time. Communicate that postpartum depression is a medical condition that requires support and understanding.

4. **Encouraging Questions:**
    - **Welcoming Inquiries:** Encourage partners and family members to ask questions and seek clarification about postpartum depression. This helps dispel misconceptions and ensures that everyone involved has accurate information.

Involving Loved Ones in the Healing Process:

1. **Attending Therapy Together:**
    - **Couples or Family Therapy:** Think about going to therapy sessions as a couple or family. Couples or family therapy can provide a structured

environment for addressing issues, improving communication, and developing coping strategies as a unit.

2. **Participating in Supportive Activities:**
   - **Joining Supportive Activities:** Encourage partners and family members to participate in activities that promote well-being, such as exercise, mindfulness, or self-care practices. Shared activities contribute to a supportive and positive atmosphere.

3. **Assisting with Daily Tasks:**
   - **Sharing Responsibilities:** Loved ones can assist with daily tasks, including childcare, household chores, and meal preparation. Sharing responsibilities lightens the load for the individual experiencing PPD and creates a supportive environment.

4. **Providing Emotional Support:**
   - **Active Listening:** Partners and family members can provide emotional support by actively listening without judgment. This involves creating a safe space for the

individual to express their feelings and concerns.

5. **Encouraging Professional Help:**
   - **Supporting Treatment Plans:** Loved ones can play a crucial role in encouraging the individual to seek professional help and adhere to treatment plans. This support may involve attending therapy sessions, doctor appointments, or medication management consultations.

6. **Respecting Boundaries:**
   - **Understanding Personal Limits:** While involvement is crucial, it's also important for partners and family members to respect the individual's need for personal space and boundaries. Striking a balance between support and respecting autonomy is essential.

7. **Planning for Self-Care:**
   - **Fostering Self-Care:** Partners and family members can actively support self-care practices by assisting with childcare to allow time for relaxation, exercise, or engaging in activities that bring joy and fulfilment.

❖ Partner and family support can significantly impact the journey of healing from postpartum depression. Building a strong support network, fostering open communication, and actively involving loved ones in the healing process create an environment conducive to recovery. By working together, partners and family members can contribute to the well-being of the individual experiencing PPD and promote a healthier family dynamic.

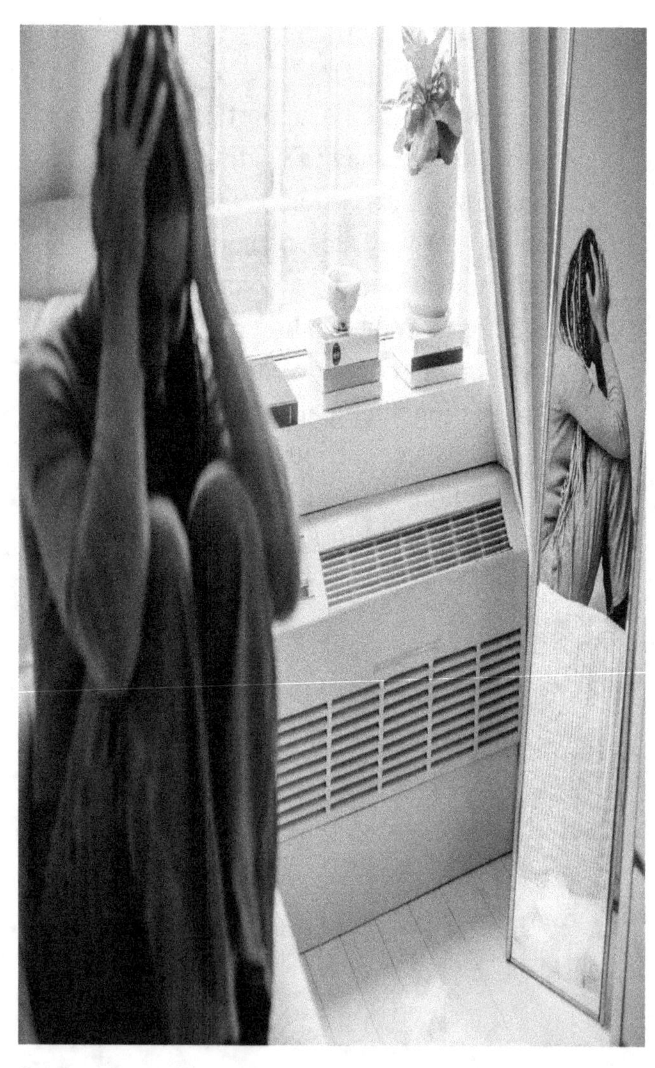

Chapter Ten

Postpartum Depression and Breastfeeding

As nursing moms manage the delicate balance between their mental health and their infants' nutritional demands, postpartum depression (PPD) can present particular complications. It's important to address these considerations to ensure the well-being of both the mother and the baby.

Considerations for Breastfeeding Mothers:

1. **Consultation with Healthcare Providers:**
   - **Open Communication:** Breastfeeding mothers experiencing PPD should maintain open communication with their healthcare providers. Discussing mental health concerns, including symptoms and treatment options, is crucial for developing a comprehensive care plan.
2. **Medication Considerations:**
   - **Medication Safety:** When considering medication to treat

postpartum depression, healthcare professionals should examine how safe the drug is for nursing moms. Some antidepressants are compatible with breastfeeding, and alternative options may be explored.

3. **Monitoring Milk Supply:**
   - **Effect on Milk Production:** The quantity of milk produced may be impacted by the stress and anxiety associated with postpartum depression. Monitoring the baby's growth and consulting with a lactation consultant or healthcare provider can address concerns about breastfeeding effectiveness.

Balancing Mental Health and Infant Nutrition:

1. **Nutritional Impact on Breast Milk:**
   - **Maintaining a Balanced Diet:** Breastfeeding mothers with PPD should strive to maintain a balanced and nutritious diet. Nutrient-rich foods contribute to overall well-being and can positively impact the nutritional content of breast milk.

2. **Hydration and Self-Care:**
   - **Adequate Hydration:** Staying hydrated is crucial for breastfeeding mothers. Proper self-care, including adequate sleep and regular meals, supports both mental health and the production of breast milk.
3. **Pumping and Milk Storage:**
   - **Creating Flexibility:** For mothers who may need to take medication or attend therapy sessions, pumping breast milk and storing it allows for flexibility in feeding the baby while prioritizing the mother's mental health.
4. **Support from Family and Partners:**
   - **Assistance with Infant Care:** Partners and family members can provide support by assisting with infant care responsibilities, allowing the breastfeeding mother time for self-care and rest.
5. **Involving a Lactation Consultant:**
   - **Addressing Breastfeeding Challenges:** A lactation consultant can help breastfeeding mothers address any challenges they may encounter, such as latching difficulties or concerns about milk

supply. Seeking professional guidance can enhance the breastfeeding experience.

6. **Supplementation and Alternative Feeding Options:**
   - **Exploring Options:** In certain situations, supplementation with formula or exploring alternative feeding options may be considered. This decision should be made in consultation with healthcare providers and lactation experts to ensure the infant's nutritional needs are met.

7. **Prioritizing Mental Health:**
   - **Recognizing the Importance of Self-Care:** Recognizing the importance of mental health is essential. Mothers should prioritize self-care, seek professional help for postpartum depression, and understand that maintaining mental well-being is vital for providing quality care to their infants.

❖ Balancing postpartum depression and breastfeeding involves careful consideration of both the mental health needs of the mother and the nutritional needs of the infant. Open communication with healthcare providers, prioritizing self-care, and seeking support from partners and family members are crucial steps in navigating this delicate balance. By addressing these considerations, breastfeeding mothers can work towards achieving a harmonious and supportive environment for both themselves and their infants.

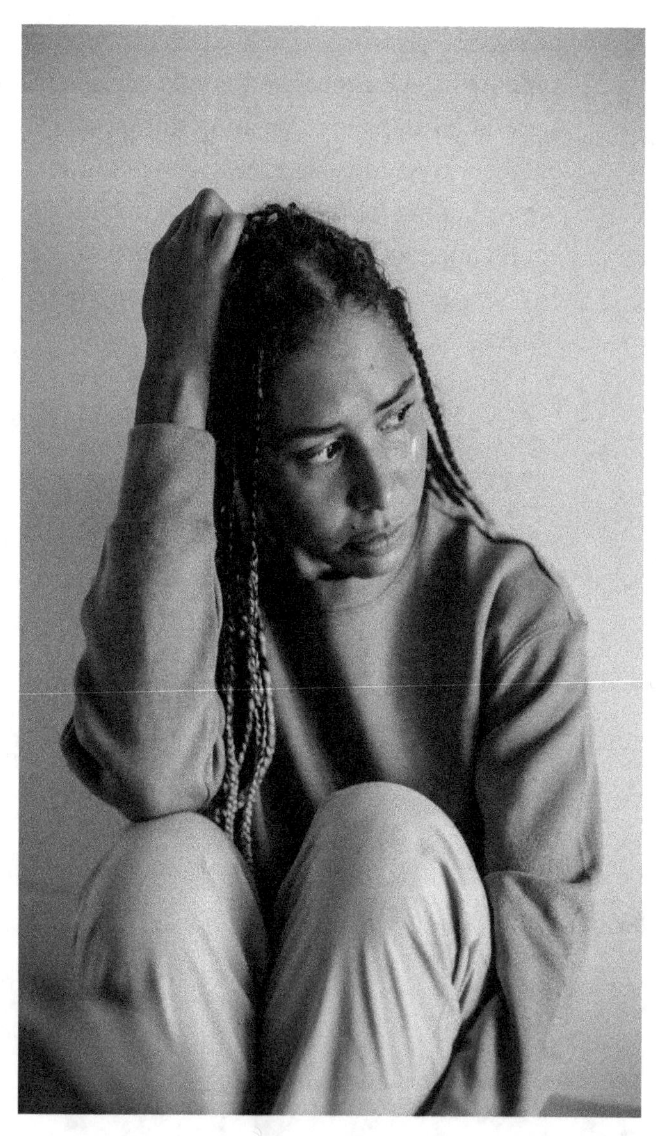

Chapter Eleven

Preventive Measures

Preventive measures play a crucial role in addressing postpartum depression (PPD) by identifying and managing risk factors and proactively planning for the postpartum period. Recognizing these factors and implementing preventive strategies can contribute to the well-being of both mothers and infants.

Recognizing and Addressing Risk Factors:

1. **Personal and Family History:**
   - **Assessment and Monitoring:** Women with a personal or family history of depression or mental health conditions are at an increased risk of developing PPD. Recognizing this risk and monitoring for early signs during the postpartum period is crucial.
2. **Previous Episodes of Depression:**
   - **Preventive Interventions:** Women who have experienced depression

before becoming pregnant or during previous pregnancies should be identified early in prenatal care. Preventive interventions, such as counselling and support, can be implemented proactively.

3. **Stressful Life Events:**
   - **Anticipatory Guidance:** Identifying and addressing stressful life events during pregnancy allows for anticipatory guidance. Providing resources and support to cope with potential stressors, such as financial concerns or relationship issues, can help prevent the onset of PPD.

4. **Lack of Social Support:**
   - **Creating a Network of Support:** Postpartum depression is more common in women who receive insufficient social support. Encouraging the development of a strong support system, including partners, family, and friends, is vital for preventive measures.

5. **Complications During Pregnancy or Birth:**
   - **Early Intervention:** Complications during pregnancy or birth can contribute to PPD. Early

intervention, including counselling
and support, can help women
navigate the emotional impact of
these experiences.

Postpartum Planning and Education:

1. **Prenatal Education Programs:**
   - **Educating pregnant Mothers:** It is
     beneficial for pregnant mothers and
     their partners to learn about
     postpartum mental health in prenatal
     education programs, as it can help
     them recognize and address any
     issues that may arise, and seek
     support if needed.
2. **Postpartum Care Plans:**
   - **Developing Personalized Plans:**
     Healthcare providers can work with
     expectant mothers to develop
     personalized postpartum care plans
     that address risk factors and provide
     resources for mental health support.
3. **Screening and Monitoring:**
   - **Routine Mental Health Screening:**
     Incorporating routine mental health
     screening during prenatal and
     postpartum appointments allows for

early identification of risk factors and symptoms. This enables timely intervention and support.

4. **Partner Involvement:**
   - **Educating Partners:** Including partners in postpartum education helps create a supportive environment. Partners can play a crucial role in recognizing signs of PPD, encouraging help-seeking behaviour, and providing emotional support.

5. **Access to Mental Health Resources:**
   - **Providing Information and Resources:** Ensure that expectant mothers are aware of available mental health resources, including counselling services, support groups, and hotlines. Having this information readily available can facilitate timely access to support.

6. **Encouraging Self-Care Practices:**
   - **Promoting Well-Being:** Educating expectant mothers on the importance of self-care practices, including adequate sleep, proper nutrition, and stress management, contributes to overall well-being and may act as preventive measures.

7. **Postpartum Follow-Up Care:**
    - **Continuity of Care:** Establishing postpartum follow-up care ensures ongoing support and monitoring. It allows healthcare providers to assess the emotional well-being of new mothers and intervene if signs of PPD arise.

❖ Postpartum depression prevention entails a multimodal strategy that includes identifying and managing risk factors, offering guidance and assistance during pregnancy, and creating postpartum care plans. By implementing these measures, healthcare providers and support systems can work collaboratively to create a supportive environment that promotes the mental health and well-being of new mothers.

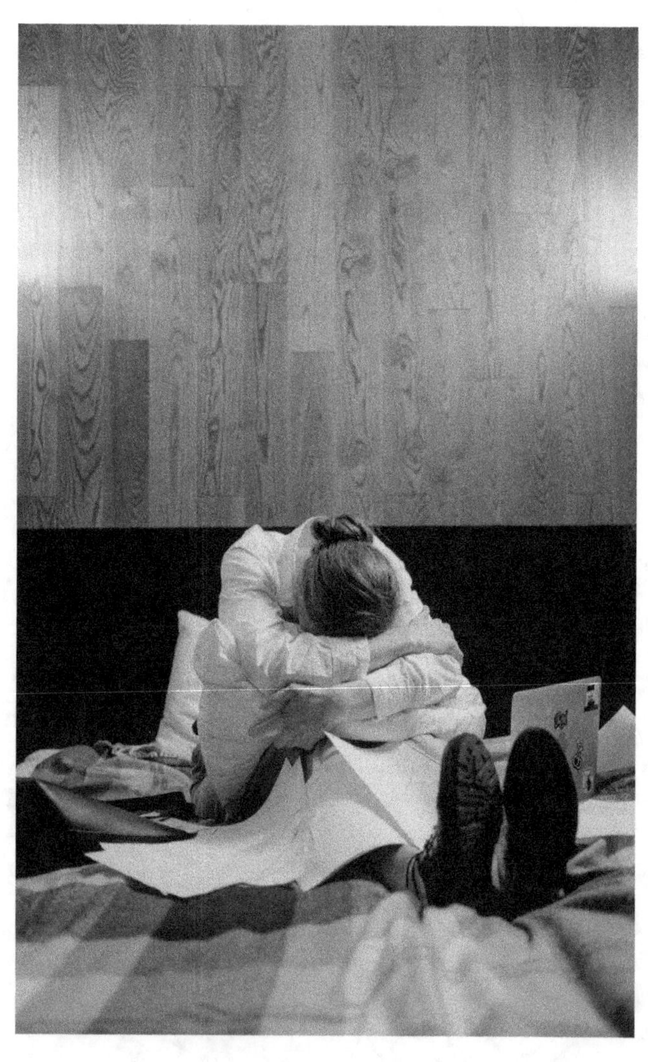

Chapter Twelve

Coping Strategies for Daily Life

Postpartum depression (PPD) must be managed through the application of practical daily practices that assist in stress management, responsibility balancing, and self-care prioritization. Here are key coping strategies for individuals experiencing PPD:

Time Management and Prioritizing Tasks:

1. **Create Realistic Schedules:**
   - Develop daily schedules that are realistic and achievable. Break tasks into manageable steps, and recognize that it's okay if everything is not completed in one day.
2. **Prioritize Self-Care:**
   - Schedule regular self-care activities, even if they are brief. This could include moments of relaxation, a short walk, or time for personal

hobbies. Prioritizing self-care contributes to overall well-being.

3. **Set Realistic Expectations:**
   - Adjust expectations and accept that there will be days when certain tasks may need to take a back seat. Setting realistic expectations prevents feelings of guilt and inadequacy.

4. **Delegate Responsibilities:**
   - Enlist the support of family members, friends, or a partner in sharing responsibilities. Delegating tasks such as childcare, household chores, or errands helps lighten the load.

5. **Use Time Blocks:**
   - Break the day into time blocks and allocate specific periods for different activities. This structured approach can help manage time more efficiently and reduce feelings of overwhelm.

Balancing Responsibilities:

1. **Communicate Openly:**
   - Communicate with your partner, family members, or friends about

your needs and limitations. Open communication fosters understanding and ensures that everyone is on the same page regarding responsibilities.

2. **Share Parenting Duties:**

    ·   Involve your partner in parenting duties. Share responsibilities such as feeding, changing diapers, and soothing the baby. A sense of shared responsibility is fostered by this cooperative approach.

3. **Establish Routines:**
    o   Establishing daily routines provides structure and predictability. Routines can be comforting for both the parent and the baby, making it easier to manage daily tasks.

4. **Learn to Say No:**
    o   Recognize your limits and be comfortable saying no to additional responsibilities or commitments. Prioritizing your mental health and well-being is crucial during the postpartum period.

5. **Utilize Support Systems:**

o Lean on your support systems, including family and friends. Express your thoughts and worries, and don't be afraid to seek assistance when you need it. Building a strong support network contributes to a more balanced and manageable daily life.

6. **Practice Mindfulness:**
   o Incorporate mindfulness practices into your daily routine. Mindfulness can help manage stress and bring attention to the present moment, reducing feelings of being overwhelmed by past or future tasks.

7. **Seek Professional Help:**
   o If feelings of stress and overwhelm persist, consider seeking professional help. A mental health professional can provide coping strategies and support tailored to your specific situation.

❖ Developing workable coping mechanisms for everyday life is part of postpartum depression management. Time management, prioritizing self-care, and balancing responsibilities are essential components of this coping process. By using these techniques and getting help when necessary, people may deal with postpartum depression's difficulties and try to lead healthier, more balanced lives daily. Top of Form

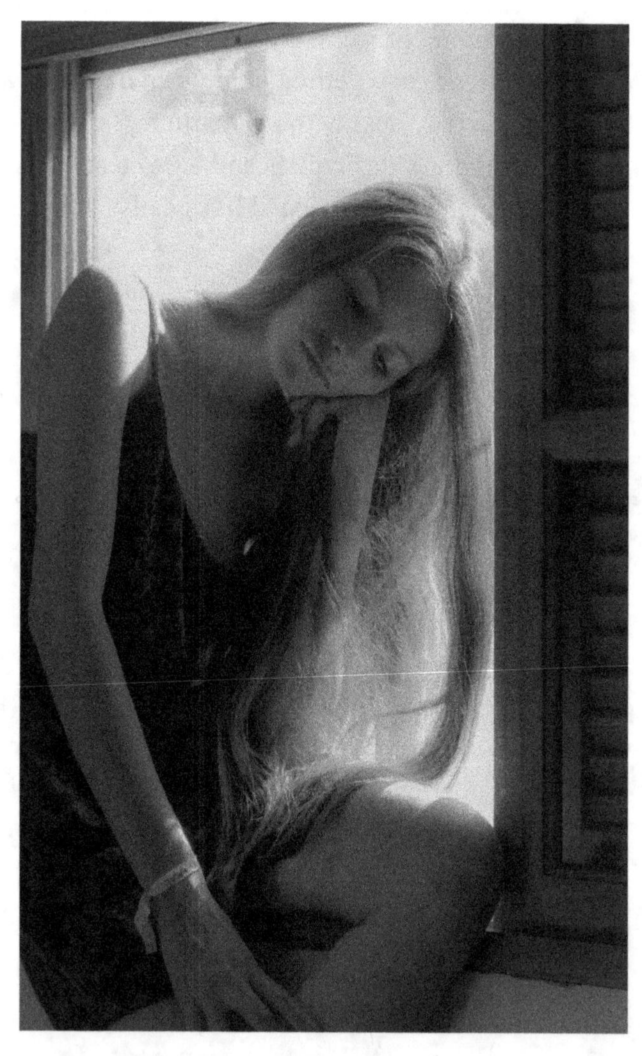

Chapter Thirteen

Building Resilience

Building resilience is crucial for individuals facing challenges, including those experiencing postpartum depression (PPD). Resilience involves developing the ability to bounce back from adversity, cope with stress, and adapt to changing circumstances. Here are key aspects of building resilience, particularly in the context of emotional well-being and finding joy in everyday moments:

Developing Emotional Resilience:

1. **Cultivating a Positive Mindset:**
   - Foster a positive outlook by consciously focusing on positive aspects of life. Challenge negative thoughts and replace them with affirmations and constructive perspectives.
2. **Practicing Mindfulness:**
   - Practice mindfulness to maintain present-moment awareness. Mindfulness involves paying attention to thoughts and feelings

without judgment. Techniques such as deep breathing and meditation can enhance emotional resilience.

3. **Building Emotional Awareness:**
   - Develop an understanding of your emotions and their triggers. Recognize when you are feeling overwhelmed and practice self-compassion. Identifying and acknowledging emotions is the first step in building emotional resilience.

4. **Cultivating Adaptive Coping Strategies:**
   - Identify and adopt healthy coping strategies that work for you. This may include seeking support from loved ones, engaging in creative activities, or practising relaxation techniques.

5. **Seeking Professional Support:**
   - Seek advice from mental health specialists. Therapy can provide tools and coping mechanisms tailored to your specific needs, promoting emotional resilience and well-being.

6. **Developing Problem-Solving Skills:**
   - Enhance your ability to address challenges by developing problem-solving skills. Break down

problems into manageable steps and approach them systematically.

Finding Joy in Everyday Moments:

1. **Practicing Gratitude:**
   - Acknowledge and value the good things in your life to help you develop a thankful attitude. Regularly expressing gratitude can shift your focus towards joy and fulfilment.
2. **Celebrating Small Achievements:**
   - Recognize and celebrate small victories and achievements. Whether it's completing a task or overcoming a challenge, acknowledging these accomplishments contributes to a sense of joy and accomplishment.
3. **Engaging in Activities You Enjoy:**
   - Schedule time for enjoyable and restorative pursuits. Whether it's reading, listening to music, or spending time in nature, engaging in enjoyable activities contributes to overall well-being.
4. **Connecting with Loved Ones:**

- Foster connections with friends and family. Share moments of joy and engage in activities together. Social connections provide emotional support and enhance the experience of positive moments.

5. **Mindful Parenting:**
   - Practice mindful parenting by fully engaging in and savouring moments with your child. Focus on the sights, sounds, and emotions of the present moment, fostering a deeper connection and joy in the parent-child relationship.

6. **Creating a Positive Environment:**
   - Surround yourself with positivity. Decorate your living space with things that bring joy, such as uplifting artwork or meaningful mementoes. A positive environment can contribute to a more positive mindset.

7. **Setting Realistic Expectations:**
   - Manage expectations and recognize that joy can be found in small, everyday moments. Setting realistic expectations reduces pressure and allows for a greater appreciation of life's simple pleasures.

❖   Building resilience involves both developing emotional strength and finding joy in everyday moments. By practising mindfulness, cultivating a positive mindset, and engaging in activities that bring joy, individuals can enhance their ability to cope with challenges and navigate the complexities of postpartum depression more effectively. Building resilience is an ongoing process that empowers individuals to embrace life's ups and downs with greater strength and optimism.

Chapter Fourteen

Conclusion

In conclusion, postpartum depression (PPD) is a challenging and complex experience that can deeply impact individuals and their families. However, it's important to recognize that with the right support, interventions, and self-care strategies, there is hope for recovery and a brighter future.

Encouragement and Hope:

1. **Seeking Help is a Sign of Strength:**
   - Seeking help is a recognition of the need for support and a commitment to one's well-being.
2. **Comprehensive Treatment is Effective:**
   - Emphasize the effectiveness of a comprehensive treatment approach. Postpartum depression can be managed holistically by combining professional assistance, including therapy or medication, with self-help techniques, social support, and lifestyle modifications.
3. **Progress is Gradual and Valuable:**
   - Recovery from postpartum depression is a gradual process. Each

step forward, no matter how small, is
a valuable achievement. Celebrate
the progress made, and remember
that healing occurs at its own pace.

Moving Forward After Postpartum Depression:

1. **Ongoing Self-Care is Essential:**
   - Stress the importance of ongoing self-care. Even after the severe episode of postpartum depression has passed, it is crucial to prioritize mental wellness through self-care strategies. Regularly check in with emotions, engage in activities that bring joy, and maintain a support network.
2. **Building a Supportive Network:**
   - Encourage individuals to continue building and maintaining a supportive network. Connections with loved ones, friends, support groups, and healthcare professionals provide ongoing encouragement and assistance in the journey forward.
3. **Learning from the Experience:**

- Reflect on the experience of postpartum depression as an opportunity for growth and self-discovery. The insights gained during this challenging time can contribute to increased resilience and a deeper understanding of oneself.

4. **Parenting with Compassion:**
    - Approach parenting with compassion and patience. Recognize that every parent faces challenges, and it is okay to seek assistance when needed. Learning to balance responsibilities and prioritize one's well-being contributes to a healthier family dynamic.

5. **Setting Realistic Expectations:**
    - Set realistic expectations for the post-recovery period. Understand that life may still have its ups and downs, and it is okay to ask for help when needed. Setting achievable goals promotes a sense of accomplishment and reduces pressure.

6. **Maintaining Open Communication:**
    - Continue to communicate openly with partners, family members, and healthcare providers. Sharing

thoughts, concerns, and
achievements fosters a supportive
environment and helps in navigating
the ongoing journey of parenting and
mental health.

Final Words:

Postpartum depression is a challenging chapter, but
it is not the entirety of the parenting journey. With
encouragement, support, and a commitment to
well-being, individuals can move forward,
embracing the joys and challenges of parenthood
with resilience and hope. Every step taken toward
healing is a testament to strength, and the future
holds the promise of brighter, more fulfilling days.
Keep in mind that there is hope and opportunity for
a successful life following postpartum depression
on the journey ahead, and you are not alone.

www.ingramcontent.com/pod-product-compliance
Lightning Source LLC
Chambersburg PA
CBHW061006260726
48661CB00005B/2084